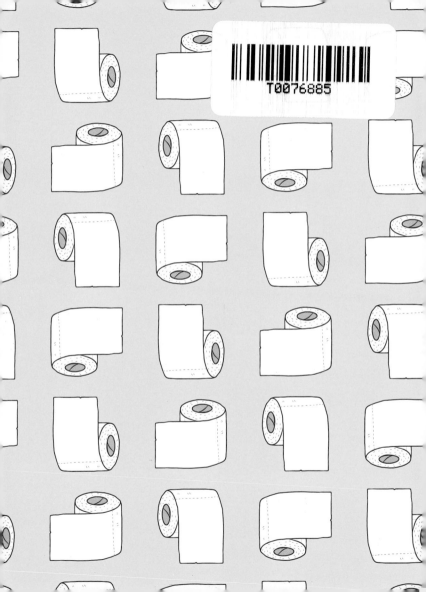

T0076885

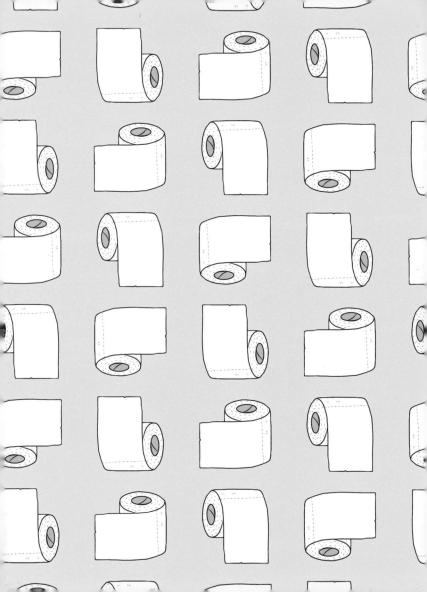

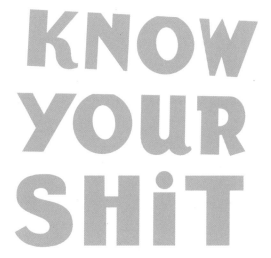

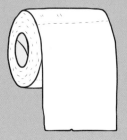

Know Your Shit

This is an officially licensed book by Cider Mill Press Book Publishers LLC.

13-Digit ISBN: 978-1-64643-223-3
10-Digit ISBN: 1-64643-223-1

This book may be ordered by mail from the publisher. Please include $5.99 for postage and handling. Please support your local bookseller first!

Books published by Cider Mill Press Book Publishers are available at special discounts for bulk purchases in the United States by corporations, institutions, and other organizations. For more information, please contact the publisher.

Cider Mill Press Book Publishers
"Where good books are ready for press"
PO Box 454
12 Spring Street
Kennebunkport, Maine 04046

Visit us online!
cidermillpress.com

Typography: BadTyp, Omnes

Printed in China

All vectors used under official license from Shutterstock.com.

1 2 3 4 5 6 7 8 9 0
First Edition

KNOW YOUR SHiT

WHAT YOUR CRAP iS TeLLiNG YOU

SHAWN SHAFNeR
Founder of The POOP Project

Illustrations by Rebecca Pry

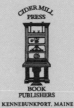

CIDER MILL PRESS

BOOK PUBLISHERS
KENNEBUNKPORT, MAINE

DEDICATION

For my parents and family: I hope this makes up for all those clogged toilets.

Thanks also to my azizam Fareed and so, so many dear friends whose persistent support, encouragement, and faith have made this possible. Lastly, thanks to all who patiently listened while I proselytized poop. That now means you, too.

CONTENTS

WHY FECAL MATTERS

I'M A POOPER.
YES, IT'S TRUE.
WE'RE ALL POOPERS.
YES, WE DOO.

From *An Inconvenient Poop*, 2015

HEY THERE, POOPER. Yes, you! Now, I know, you might not normally think of yourself that way. You hope people will notice your beautiful eyes, your rock-hard abs, or your sparkling personality. But the truth is, you are most definitely a pooper. All people, and all beings, are! Yet we generally pretend otherwise.

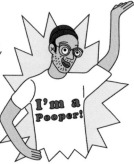

Not me. My name is Shawn Shafner, and I'm a proud pooper. Back in 2010, I created The People's Own Organic Power Project, or The POOP Project. Our mission is to foster a more loving relationship with our bodies, planet, and global community starting from the bottom up. Since our inception, I've spread my own cheeky brand of poop positivity all over the world, from the mountains of

Rwanda to the floor of the United Nations for the inaugural World Toilet Day.

But it wasn't always this way. As a kid, I was what *Poop Culture* author Dave Praeger calls "a shameful shitter." I was embarrassed to poop—especially in public—so I held it in, for hours, for days. When I finally did go, sometimes the poop was so big it would clog the toilet, and I'd be so embarrassed, and the cycle would begin again. Eventually, I realized that my shyness was constipating me. All I had to do to break the chains was poop! Slowly, I got more comfortable going when I needed to; it was far better than the alternative.

Years later, I started to research. I wanted to know my shit and understand what had happened all those years back. I read Dave's book and many, many others. I spoke with experts, toured wastewater treatment plants, and went on fecal field expeditions around the world. I saw how the shame I had expressed as a child was not really mine, but my society's. I also realized that this issue was way bigger than me: poop is kind of a big deal. Because all people and all beings do it on any good day, it's basically at the center of everything.

Now, I think it's unimaginable that we know so little about something so important to our daily functioning. How did something so ordinary get to be so obscured that English speakers don't even have a neutral term with which to speak of it? And with this most basic human experience suffused under a cone of social silence, how do we even know what normal is? Even more, how can we imagine a world that would cater to the reality of our bodies, stuck on a finite planet with a lot of other bodies? In other words, how are we supposed to fix all the super-complex problems in our world if we don't even know shit about shit?

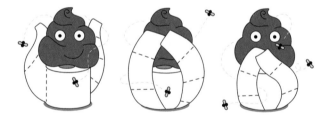

Lucky for you, dear pooper, you're already on your way to becoming excrementally enlightened. Page by page, we'll lift the lid off the potty taboo and break the stall doors down in search of the Perfect Poo. Along the way, we'll learn what happens inside your body to make poo, how the process can go wrong, and simple fixes to make sure you stay in the Goldiplops Zone. You'll also find Golden Nuggets and Pro Pooper Tips sprinkled throughout to help you look beyond the toilet bowl and understand how poop can help us save humanity.

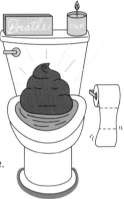

So saddle up with a nice high-fiber snack and walk—don't get the runs—to join a movement pushing for change from the bottom up! We'll see you on the other side.

♠

Shawn

> While I am an expert, I am not a doctor. What's worse, I'm talking to you through a static book; we can't even have a conversation! If you're managing major bowel distress, or simply interested in learning more, please consult diverse sources, explore through your own experience, and see a healer or medical doctor who can help you in real time.

CHAPTER ONE

TURD
AS OLD AS
TIME

PEOPLE HAVE BEEN pooping ever since they emerged on the planet. In fact, poop may be as old as the planet itself. Dinosaurs pooped; we have their fossilized turds, or coprolites, to prove it. Well before reptiles had evolved their digestive tract, however, single-celled organisms were happily eating and crapping from the same hole. In other words, poop is even older than buttholes. And every living creature today—plants, mammals, even some of those same ancient bacteria—live in a cycle of give-and-take with their ecosystem. Nutrients enter the organism, are processed and integrated, and a by-product comes back out.

Here is where things get really exciting: what looks like poop to one regurgitating, single-celled organism looks like gourmet chow to the next one in line. The earth's ecosystems rely on this nutrient recycling, as food becomes poop and poop becomes food. The amount of whale feces in the ocean, for example, directly correlates to the health of the entire aquatic food web. That's because phytoplankton feed on all that Moby Dung, which in turn feeds the rest of the ocean—including krill, the whale's favorite food. The whole world follows this model of a self-replenishing banquet. All of nature's creatures find their places, all of us connected in cycles of consumption and production.

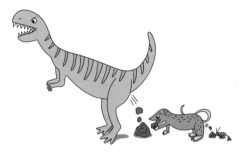

We humans often feel removed from this process. We certainly don't think of ourselves as eating poop, and a bunch of hungry bugs and microorganisms feasting on our poop is truly the stuff of nightmares. But that is actually what's happening in a septic tank, wastewater treatment plant, or hole in the woods. Poop goes in, organisms eat it, and they poop out fertilizer or become it themselves. The same is true for animal dung, as insects and bacteria transform that shit into the black gold farmers call "manure." Follow your food back to its origins, and there's always poop in there somewhere. In that way, it's kind of like magic. Like a virtuous human centipede filled with happy farm creatures.

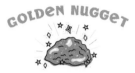

FRee RaNGe SHiTTiNG

"Life is a mystery," Madonna famously sang. "Everyone must stand alone." That might be true, but you needn't stand, sit, or squat alone when it comes to pooping. Really! Ancient Romans built public bathhouses with large, communal toilet rooms. There you could shoot the shit while you shat and bonded with your neighbors, taking turns cleaning with a vinegar-soaked sponge on a stick.

Many medieval elites pooped side by side in castle loos, called garderobes because the smell of old pee was thought to deter moths from eating the fine clothes that were stored there. One might imagine the stink also deterred people from using it, but for much of human history, people accepted that piss and shit smelled like, well, piss and shit. That's not to say they liked it, but it wasn't a shameful, private secret. Even George Washington shared a three-holer with friends at Mount Vernon. You can still see (and sometimes use) multi-seat outhouses in the United States, and the internet is littered with tourists traumatized from using open, trough-style toilets still found in China today. Like a virgin no more.

Don't get me wrong: we don't eat straight poop. And if you do favor a spoonful every now and again, as the Protestant reformer Martin Luther was said to have done, please be careful. One's own poop is more or less innocuous to ingest, but bacteria from someone else's BM can make you very sick. Even a tiny amount from unwashed hands, or from a fly that lands on a poop and then on your food, can cause serious illness and discomfort. So please, don't eat poop. And if you've really got a hankering for coprophagy (the fancy word for eating crap), go for something that just tastes like shit. Say, durian fruit, or your mother-in-law's meat loaf.

Despite these warnings, however, the fact is that we sort of eat poop all of the time. This might seem surprising because most food, like an apple, or a steak, is definitely not poop, right? But speaking broadly, much of what we eat sits somewhere along the food-to-poop-to-food pipeline. Trees expel some of their wastes into fruits and nuts. Meat may contain hormones and bodily acids left over from processes interrupted at the moment of slaughter. Some foods put us even closer to the receiving end of another being's output. The delicious squish of a good bread comes from air pockets created by yeast tooting into the dough. When that yeast's cousin feeds on sugary water, it pees out that expensive bottle of wine, craft IPA, or dry martini. Fermented foods like pickles, yogurt, and, to some degree, even coffee all follow this model: your dinner bowl is bacteria's toilet bowl. And that's just the cycle of life. L'chaim!

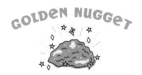

GOLDEN NUGGET

ORIGIN OF FECES

Our modern lives have obscured the important role that poop plays in our ecosystem. However, various cultures throughout history and around the world have understood this relationship. They've even told creation myths that recognize poop's contribution as a foundational building block of existence. The Kokori people of India tell tales of how our earth was pooped out by a worm. In the Arctic, the Chukchi describe how life emerged from Raven's droppings as he flew across the sky.

In Tanzania, the Wapangwa explain how ants devoured their own dung pile and pooped it out again, slowly building the mound we live on. Even Abrahamic religions may reference our excremental origins. The first person is created from the earth—in Hebrew, *adamah*—which lends its name to the earthling *Adam*. From the dust we come, and to the dust we go. Give us this day our daily whole grain bread that this, too, shall pass easily into dust.

CHAPTER TWO

THE
PERFECT
POOP

THE FOUNTAIN OF YOUTH. The Holy Grail.
The Perfect Poop.

Do you, dear pooper, dare to seek? Shrouded in mystery, sought after since antiquity, many have tried to obtain the Perfect Poop. Yet in striving—in straining—they fail.

Many others doubt that such a thing really exists. They call the Perfect Poop a myth, a fool's errand, a battle with sulfuric windmills. But I've seen it. I've been down to the depths of our entrails and lived to tell the tale.

Are you ready for it?

Actually, I'm not sure you are. Would you even know it if you saw it? It could be right under your seat at this very moment! Would you recognize it?

Many people don't look at their poo. This is their first mistake. Friends, let me say it again in big letters:

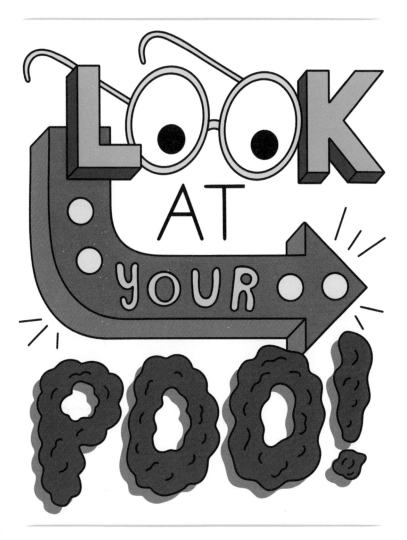

That singular, stinking sensation is a gift from your body. Once you've learned what to look for, checking your poop can be like looking inside yourself. Like sticking a telescope up your bum, but way more hygienic and much less invasive.

Your poop is also, well, a piece of shit. It's a mere messenger from our insides, silent and powerless. If we want to change what we see on the outside, we have to start from within.

The truth is, there is no one Perfect Poop. As with the rest of our human experience, diversity is the norm. Some people have big poops. Some people have little poops. Some people poop three times a day, and others poop three times a week. Each poop your body makes is a direct response to the food you ingested, your particular physiology, your nutritional needs, your gut microflora, and your individual life circumstances (stress, sleep, physical activity) during digestion.

Now, let us hold these poos to be self-evident; not all are created equal. Doctors break poops down into seven ranked categories called the Bristol Stool Chart.

Here, we make things even easier using the Goldiplops Zone model. That is: some are too dry; some are too wet; some are just right. But as for your perfect poo? The only way to find out is to venture deep into this dark matter, where few have gone before.

Isn't this fun? Feel free to bring a cardboard sword. And watch out for the splash zone!

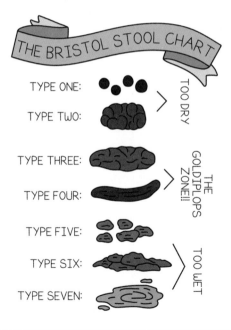

THE BRISTOL STOOL CHART

TYPE ONE:
TYPE TWO:
} TOO DRY

TYPE THREE:
TYPE FOUR:
} THE GOLDIPLOPS ZONE!!

TYPE FIVE:
TYPE SIX:
TYPE SEVEN:
} TOO WET

WHAT'S iN A POOP?

The philosopher René Descartes famously said, "I think, therefore I am." Thoughts are fine and good, but the 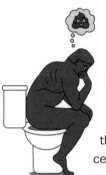 thick brown goop we leave behind is the tangible evidence of our embodied existence. A poop is obviously distinct and set apart from the pooper who pooped it. Yet, for some time, they were an indistinct, intertwined entity. And even though the little turd has now been eviscerated from the owner's body, it still contains DNA, dead cells, and living bacteria that now exist independently, sent out into the world like pigs to make their fortune. (Beware little turd: only the brick shithouse can keep you safe!)

Poop's liminal nature is one reason that many societies have revered shit as a source of magic, miracle cures, or curses. It is both of us and separate from us. Of the body and of the world. Your shit is your responsibility while it's in you, but becomes the collective's responsibility once it emerges. Looking at your poop is like looking at yourself in a mirror; it reflects some essential quality, but it's not really you at all.

Like the rest of you, your poop is mostly water. This may seem surprising, since we normally think of a number two as solid waste. But if you removed all the water from a year's worth of pee and poo, there would actually be twice as many solids in the pee. (Proving once again why it's number one.) Drain the water from a turd, and 75 percent of it washes away. Exactly what constitutes the remaining 25 percent depends on your diet: fibrous fruits and veggies, meats, and highly processed foods all influence the solid material in any particular poop. After the water has been expelled, poop's remaining contents are roughly:

- 25 to 54 percent living and dead microbes from your gut, including bacteria, viruses, yeast, and archaea (microbes that exclusively inhabit extreme environments)

- 25 percent carbohydrates and the fiber your grandma used to call "roughage"

- 2 to 25 percent nitrogen-rich, undigested protein from food, and from bacterial and intestinal cells shed during digestion

- 2 to 15 percent fat, mostly from diet

What's left includes salts and minerals like calcium and iron phosphate, the remains of digestive juices that help give poop its color, and mucus. Microplastics have also become evident in our poop as humans become ever more reliant on plastic food and water packaging. For better or for worse, we truly are what we eat. And what we leave behind.

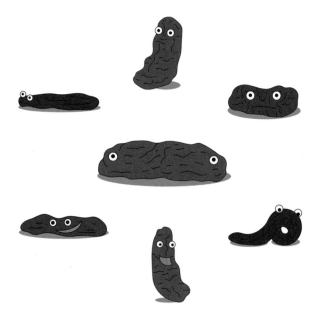

CHAPTER THREE

KEEPING A LOG LOG

OUR TURDS ARE ALWAYS spilling the tea, but
few of us know how to listen. We think shit is just shit,
like all penguins are like all other penguins. Sure, we can
see that some are bigger, some smaller, some have little
tufts of orange hair coming out of their ears. Is it black
and white? Does it waddle? Is it a bird? Okay, I got it,
it's a penguin—let's get on with our lives already! But by
paying a little bit of attention each day, you could easily
learn to identify each species, where it comes from,
what unique abilities it possesses, and whether a particular penguin is looking peppy or pooping out.

So, too, with a little observation, can you get to know
your shit. A minute's observation will do. What's the
shape? Is it really wet, really dry, or in the middle? Does
it have a distinguishing color? Is it particularly yellow,
green, or dark? Does it have a distinguishing smell—particularly shitty, strangely inoffensive, or miraculously
sweet? Can you see any evidence of what you ate in it?

This last question is particularly helpful, especially when
beginning a log log. Whatever poop your body produces
is in direct relationship to the food that proffered it.
Something your body "disagreed with" might look and

feel like a dark and stormy night, while an agreeable meal often comes out looking and feeling fresh as a summer day. Understanding the relationship between food and poo is key to decoding your doo-doo's dialogue on diet.

Poop is a messy messenger and, like most of us, not always clear in its communication style. While it's responding directly to your food, it's also a complicated amalgamation of your entire digesting being, including your overall health, mental wellness, sleep, and so much more. Let's say, for example, that you order pasta pomodoro on a hot date.

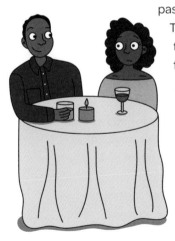

The next day, shit gets real. The toilet might look like a mud fight because you're allergic to gluten, or it might be because that date scared you shitless. Tracking our bowel response over time can help us isolate variables and connect the dots so the picture becomes clear. Maybe we need to avoid gluten *and* take a Xanax.

Only regular observation can tell you what is "regular" for you.

Let's get started! Grab a teeny note-book, a clipboard you can hang on a pin by the potty, or order a journal or phone app made for this purpose. Exactly what information you want to track will depend on your needs and, frankly, how anal you want to be.

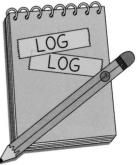

For me, I take a small notebook and make four columns, labeling them at the top: "time," "input," "output," and "notes." I record events in the order that they hap-pened; since I rarely eat and poop at the same time, the time column is steady while the other two alternate. I make any special notes about how I felt while eating: for example, "maybe ate too much," or "felt very satisfied." After bowel movements, I note anything extraordinary: shape, moisture, color, if things passed smoothly and evenly or only through struggle and strain.

It takes the average body twenty-four to seventy-two hours to complete the food-to-poo journey, so most people can begin to correlate their results in just a few days. I like to draw lines connecting meals to poops—or sometimes circles, if I notice a meal dropped as a deuce or further divided. Especially when getting started, make things easy for yourself by throwing in a few clear markers. Beets, corn, or quinoa, anyone? With greater awareness of the food-to-poop relationship, you'll soon be able to sniff out even less obvious evidence. No shit, Sherlock!

Now that I've got all of the evidence, I can look for patterns. This is how I realized that popcorn comes back out of me as a satisfied, bulky log, and that I always have an anxious poop before going onstage. Becoming mindful of our bowel movements can not only help us find a diet that promotes our singular body's singular needs, but it can also help us create a life that supports our ideal wellness, too.

There's no wrong way to keep a log log. Find what works for you! I wipe while sitting and check the toilet before closing the lid and flushing. (Seriously, folks. Close the lid and avoid spraying billions of tiny poop particles around your bathroom.) Then I wash my hands and make brief notes about the day's inputs and outputs so far. Someone who stands to wipe—you know who you are—might take notes before cleaning. And anyone using a bidet is already winning at life, so keeping a food and stool diary is a bonus. Even if you don't keep a journal, checking the toilet every time you go is a helpful litmus test on whether things are generally working, or clogging up the works. It's not a big deal; it's just shit! The most important thing is that you have a loving relationship with the body you call home.

CHAPTER FOUR

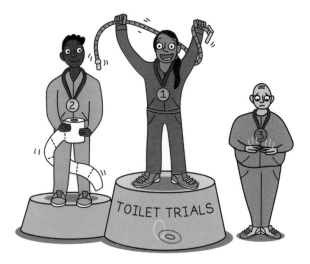

TOILETS AND TOILET PAPER

WATER, WATER EVERYWHERE AND NOT A DROP TO FLUSH

Water can't help but move. It flows from oceans and mountain rains to rivers and valley streams, coursing over land until it finds another ocean, or collects in rivers and ponds. Or in your toilet bowl.

The water in your toilet comes from the same place as all other household "in" flows. Shower, sink, laundry, toilet, etc., all receive water through the same, connected branch of pipes. These in turn take water from bigger pipes that we could follow upstream to a water treatment plant, and even farther up the line to reservoirs fed by rivers and rain, and the whole water cycle you learned about in school. Your mouth is at the tail end of that intake as you bring a cold glass of tap water to your lips. (You really should drink tap, by the way; it's way more strictly regulated than that bottled marketing you buy. Plus, you already pay for it in your water rates. That's hydration you can take to the bank!)

When that liquid is finished coursing through your body, you assume a new position on the toilet and at the start of water's outflow. Then flush and forget, right? What follows, however, is not happily ever after.

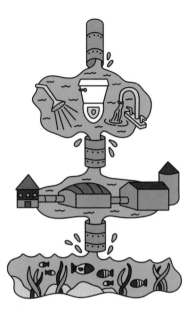

You, dear reader, are obviously above average. But if you were an average person living in the United States, almost 27 percent of the water flowing into your home would leave out the toilet. At 18.5 gallons, that's more water than any other household appliance (washing machine, shower, sink, etc.). Every year, Americans spend $5 billion to flush over 1.2 trillion gallons of clean drinking water down the toilet. That's how much money it costs to clean and transport all the water we're just going to shit in. But that figure pales in comparison to the amount of energy and chemicals it will take to separate that poop and pee back out of the water. In fact, 2 percent of electricity usage in the United States goes to transporting and treating water flows. In 2019 alone, 34 million metric tons of CO_2 were pumped into the air from processing our poop.

This story is not unique to the United States. Like a leaky lamb hot on Mary's trail, excessive water waste follows the flush toilet wherever it goes. The average Canadian uses almost 26.5 gallons to flush each day. That's the equivalent of 200 water bottles full of drinkable water—three times more water than the average person will drink that day. In the UK, the average person flushes more water each day than they drink all month, with a third of the water coming into their home leaving through the toilet. Environmentally-conscious Germans use less water overall, but still 31 percent of their home water is used for flushing. Japan has the world's most efficient flush toilets, some of which can flush your poop and wash your bum with less than a gallon per use (low flow toilets in the US use 1.6 gallons). Yet flush toilets still account for about a quarter of water usage inside the average Japanese home.

The "flush and forget" sanitation system was built for a world where water and energy supplies were inexhaustible. However, that world is quickly disappearing down the drain. According to the World Health Organization, "Water scarcity impacts 40 percent of the world's population, and as many as 700 million people are at-risk of being displaced as a result of drought by 2030." If we're not careful, we'll soon be up shit creek without a paddle, or a drop to drink.

Luckily, there are innovative solutions just around the riverbend. Greywater toilets, for example, flush with water that's already been used, like from your shower. Permaculture treatment turns your outflow into fish food and fertilizer for tropical plants. Poke and bananas, anyone? But the simplest solution is not to make a problem—that is, if we don't put the poop and pee in the water, we don't need to separate them back out.

Compost toilets (sometimes called "earth closets") safely treat pee and poo without introducing water or harsh chemicals. They produce a cleaner fertilizer than a centralized wastewater treatment plant (or "water resource recovery facility") ever could, since they don't combine with everything else going down a city's sewers. They're like the speakeasy of sewage treatment; they don't let just anybody in. Compost systems are also much more resilient in natural disasters, and waaaaaay cheaper to build and maintain.

There's also an in-between step called urine diversion. This means separating the pee into its own container before flushing or composting the poo. Sweden's been mining this liquid gold for years, as has Vermont's Rich Earth Institute, along with many others. Why? Surprisingly, pee contains most of the nutrients coming out of us, and also chemical residues from the medications we ingest. Many centralized plants do not have the advanced (and expensive) technologies needed to fully remove these fertilizers or pharmaceuticals from the water. That means they are released into our rivers and streams, where the nutrients promote toxic algae, and marine life winds up popping our pills. When urine is separated at the source, the medicines appear to be rendered harmless, and the fertilizers can go to work promoting the right plants. Try using it in your own garden in place of chemical plant foods, and let there be pee on earth!

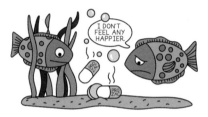

Unfortunately, compost toilets and seamless urine diversion are not yet possible for everyone, especially in dense urban environments. But there are still lots of ways to reduce your water consumption in the bathroom. Here's an easy one: embrace a pee-pee pool. On average, four out of five flushes are just for urine, which itself comprises only 1 percent of what enters a wastewater treatment plant. Flushing for poop but letting the yellow mellow could save 80 percent of the water we currently send down the drain, which means more water for all of the things we really need. I'll drink to that!

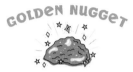

TOILETS OF THE FUTURE

There are now plenty of phone apps that make it super easy and convenient to be a poop sleuth. But is it gross to use your phone on the toilet? Maybe, but it's already happening: 88 percent of Americans sometimes use their phone on the toilet, while 46 percent admit to doing it every time. New smart toilets may relieve us of that necessity. They can take your blood pressure, send an image of your stool to an app or a doctor, and advanced models can even do a urinalysis. Dr. Loo to the rescue!

The real future of the toilet, however, is in defecatory justice. You read that right. "Defecatory justice" is a term coined by scholar and activist Sarah Nahar. In her words, "Defecatory justice materializes through designs that allow what comes out of bodies to remain within the natural cycle of decomposition . . . and is in relationship with other justice movements in service of collective liberation." Though it may seem surprising, fair access to toilets has been a major part of many liberation movements, including the fight for Indigenous autonomy, women's rights, civil rights, disability rights, rights for all genders and sexual expressions, access for house-less communities, even religious freedom. Control the toilet, and you control whose bodies can be where, and how free they are to poo, pee, and simply be.

What would these toilets of the future look like? It's likely not a one-size-fits-all model. Perhaps we haven't even imagined it yet! What we do know is that these toilets will be accessible to all, safe, clean, and ecologically resilient, with a range of features that cater to all the diverse needs of our beautiful human population. Until that day, remember to clean your devices regularly.

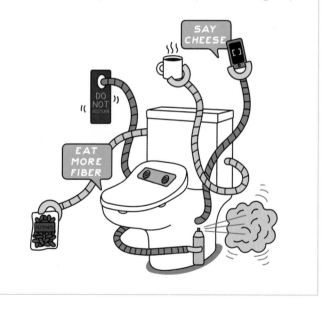

PAPER IS FOR WRITING. WATER IS FOR WASHING.

Somewhere along the process of pooping and taking notes, you'll want to clean your butt. Sure, your bowels may bless you with an immaculate delivery, but it's always better to clean preemptively than to see your error spelled out in skid marks and an itchy bum. That said, not all cleaning options are created equal.

Toilet paper was invented in China where, by the fourteenth century, it was manufactured by the millions. A new product made specifically for the purpose of anal hygiene is the exception, however, not the rule. As human history has shown, just about anything can work to get excess poop off your butt. Is it easily available, not too rough, and basically trash already? Then people have cleaned their cheeks with it. From seaweed to snow, rocks, sticks, and leaves, the natural world is our oyster shell for wiping (or scraping, as it were). Old cloth, rope, or even shards of pottery have been employed for scrubbing the pelvic floor, while corncobs and the Sears catalog were favored in American outhouses of the past.

Today's Americans, however, love toilet paper, and we are quickly spreading our enthusiasm around the world. We fold it, bunch it, and wrap it around our hands to the tune of 36.5 billion rolls a year. That's 15 million trees, 473 billion gallons of water, and 253,000 tons of chlorine bleach for whitening a paper we're just going to wipe our asses with. This, my friends, is a grave derriere error (a derri-error?). Not only is toilet paper an environmental inanity, but as far too many people's underwear will attest, it simply isn't doing the job. I mean, if I pooped on your butt, would you just wipe it off? No! First you'd punch me in the face, and then you'd take a long, hot shower.

That's why most of the sane world uses water to clean between the cheeks. For many, this brings to mind the French-style bidet, meaning "little horse" due to the way it's straddled by the user. But millions of people accomplish the same task simply by pouring water from a bottle or pitcher down their crack, manually removing debris, then washing their hands with soap. Somewhere in the middle, you can find many varieties that peek out from under the back of the toilet seat and, with the press of a button or turn of a dial, spray fresh water straight to your nockhole. While it does use water, it's far less environmentally taxing than toilet paper and you never have to buy more!

Some people will wipe for as long as they live; if that's your hill, I won't stop you from dying on it. (Though if you have a vagina, please make sure to wipe front to back, okay?) But for the sake of your own hygiene, I encourage you to use a little wetness. But be warned: WET WIPES ARE NOT FLUSHABLE. They may go down your toilet, but they don't dissolve like paper. What's worse, they bond with fats in the sewer system (like that hamburger grease you also shouldn't put down the drain) to form major clogs called "fatbergs." This is a growing problem, and one that costs cities millions of dollars to fix. Wet wipes (and kitchen grease) should always go in the trash. My recommendation? Spit on your toilet paper! Saliva doesn't clump the toilet paper like water, it provides better lubrication, and it's available wherever you are. This practice has not only improved my life on a regular basis but now, like Pavlov's dog, I salivate every time nature calls.

CHAPTER FIVE

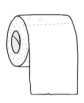

POOP FACTORY: HOW IS THE SAUSAGE MADE?

THERE COMES A TIME in every parent's life when they must answer that most uncomfortable of questions: "Mommy, where does poop come from?" If she's feeling cheeky, she might say, "It comes from your butt," and hope to end the discussion. But that's not actually true for all poopers, including anyone whose colon has been replaced with a colostomy bag. And it's an answer that will inevitably lead to more questions as the child smiles that shit-eating grin and says, "But how does poop get to your butt?" If he really tried, little Sammy could keep asking this question on a journey all the way up your butt, out your mouth, and back to the beginning of time. As you already know, every day's deposit is our own body's ode to the eternal churning of nutrients through the earth's crust.

The answer to this question, however, is of the utmost importance if we are to find the Perfect Poop. For no poo was conceived immaculately—not even holy shit. Every poo has an origin story. If we want to change the outcome, we have to understand the relationship between what went in and what's going on inside.

For the sake of this short chapter, let's agree that the moment of poo's conception coincides with consumption. In fact, digestion begins with desire. We see, smell, or even imagine something delicious (pizza or ice cream, anyone?) and our mouth begins to fill with the digestive fluid known as saliva. Check your mouth right now. If you like pizza and ice cream—or how about chili, chocolate, or fresh-baked bread?—just reading those words and imagining those treats can get your fluids flowing. Saliva's job is to act like oil in the gears, lubricating the works. It contains enzymes that begin breaking down your food, and its production signals to the rest of your digestive factory that it's time to get in gear.

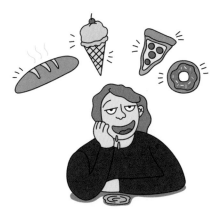

If this section has made you hungry, why not grab a snack? As Buddhist monks have long known, slowly eating even a single raisin can help us become mindful of how amazing and complex our digestive system is. Eat while you read, and tour your very own poop factory in living color!

Digestion begins with desire and ends with your daily deuce. In between head and tail, the digestive factory breaks down food into smaller and smaller particles, delivers energy and nutrients to the body, and carts away waste by-products the body cannot use. We're basically a giant worm that surrounded itself with a human body. The system even moves in a similar way. You know how a worm crawls by squeezing together and then releasing in rhythmic motions? Much of our digestive tract is built like that. It's a tube of muscles rhythmically contracting and relaxing, an action known as peristalsis, that gently moves food down and out. The tube is punctuated all along and at each end with a sphincter—a ring-shaped muscle—that protects the tube from the outside world or allows that world inside. So it turns out Wayne and Garth were right: a sphincter does say "What?"

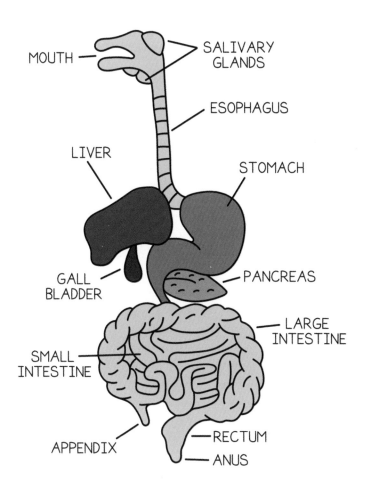

Once we consent to letting something in, our lips, teeth, jaw, and tongue work together to slice, slurp, tear, and lick food into the mashing machine between your molars. It's like the old joke: "How do you eat an elephant? One bite at a time." Until we can protract our mouths around that elephant like a python, this first stop on the slippery factory floor is where food gets small enough and wet enough to swallow. This mashed-up food, called a bolus, is now ready for the next room.

Gulp! That's the sound of a bolus passing through the upper esophageal sphincter. From there, it pulses peristaltically down the esophagus, through the lower esophageal sphincter, and into the stomach. When the bolus reaches this stretchy pouch, it floods with highly acidic digestive juices that liquify your lunch into a slurry called "chyme." The stomach's membrane is pretty amazing; it produces acid strong enough to transform your burger into a smoothie while also protecting the stomach. So while we sometimes feel hungry enough to eat our own insides, we manage not to most of the time.

Passing through another sphinctral threshold, the chyme enters the first chamber of the small intestine, where one final blast of bile and enzymes from the liver, pancreas, and gallbladder is spritzed into the brew.

Now what had been a fairly straight digestive stream becomes a winding lazy river. In order to pull all the nutrients out of the food you eat, your body needs lots of time and contact with your food. It's sort of like panning for gold. The longer you sit there, sifting water through your pan, the shinier nuggets you're bound to find. Your small intestine is narrow and quite long—about three 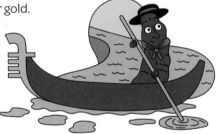 and a half times taller than you are—all coiled up inside your belly. Not only that, but the interior walls of your sausage casing are ribbed with mucosal folds and velvety villi that penetrate into the chyme to lick up every last drop of energy and nutrition. Sounds sexy, no? There's a reason that animal intestines have historically been used as condoms.

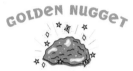

GOLDEN NUGGET

LiKe THEY DOO ON THE DiSCOVERY CHANNEL

The animal kingdom has found many ways to achieve optimal nutrition in limited space. Ruminants like cows and sheep regurgitate their food and chew it again through a system of multiple stomachs. Sloths work so hard trying to pull nutrition out of an otherwise-toxic diet that they spend up to 60 percent of their time just resting and digesting. Bunnies double the length of their digestive tract by eating their first excretion, taking a second pass at lunch, and finally hopping away from their droppings. You'll never look at Bugs's shit-eating grin the same way again.

Near the lower right side of your belly, another sphincter opens, and the small intestine empties itself into your large intestine. By now, 90 percent of what the body relates to as "food" has largely been absorbed and dispatched to your cells. What remains are tough fibers from plant life (hello, corn!), intestinal cells shed during digestion, salts or electrolytes, bile-derived pigments, and a whole lot of water. The large intestine circles your abdomen like a food waste Ferris wheel, taking your chyme on a peristaltic ride up the ascending colon on the right, across the transverse colon just under your ribs, and down the descending colon on the left side.

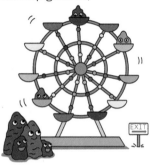

THE MIND-BODY MICROBIOME

No ride through the large intestine is complete without a visit from trillions of bacteria. That's right; not only is your poop some other organism's food, but even your pre-poop is food for the bacteria and other microorganisms that live in your gut. While it may sound creepy, it's only part of the story. In fact, your whole body is teeming with life, from anus-free *Demodex* mites that live on your skin and poop when they die to very special colonies inhabiting all your intimate, moist parts. Throughout the body, these friends work hard to co-regulate, fight off bad bacteria, and maintain your health. When gut bacteria feed off your mostly digested food, they poop out things your body needs, like vitamin K. The gut microbiome is critical to proper digestion and immune response, and it even exerts influence over your mood. Hence, we talk about a "gut feeling," and transplant technology is being developed to help restore microflora to anyone who's lost it. Perhaps most importantly, these teeny critters break down carbohydrates in the ascending colon via a process of fermentation. Fermentation's by-product? The gas we pass. So let your family dog off the hook; blame it on the biome.

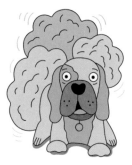

It's hard to believe it, but our tour through the factory is winding down. It's been a long journey! Depending on your diet, it takes twenty-four to seventy-two hours for what you ate as food to reappear as poop. Most of this time is spent in the large intestine, where water is slowly absorbed back into your bloodstream, transforming the slurry into a fibrous log that collects in the rectum. Here we come to our final sphincter, the anus. Like two-faced Janus, the sphincter looks both inward and outward. Our unconscious controls the inner ring, which, when feeling pressure, tells our brain that there's a package out for delivery. The outer ring is generally under conscious control, so we can choose not to shit our pants. That said, we all know how some packages can wait at the door for hours, while others demand immediate reception. Wishing you relief, however it comes, and a spare pair of underwear just in case.

Now that you and your digestive factory are better acquainted, you can take better control over product outcomes. Like any other manufacturing plant, it functions best when fed high-quality raw materials, the machines are well maintained, and the employees are happy. In the next few chapters, we'll see what happens when things go awry, and how to optimize our chances of hitting the Goldiplops Zone.

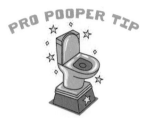

PRO POOPER TIP

TAKE A BACKWARD GLANCE: FIND YOUR ANUS

Assholes get a bad name, but this nether passageway is truly a wondrous portal. Disconnected from, or even disgusted by, this orifice, our relationship to the anus can range from neglectful to downright abusive. Like the rest of you, your butthole just wants to feel seen! Of course, that's not an easy ask. Our anus hides behind us and between our fleshy cheeks. But(t) there are good reasons to grab a mirror, bend over, and seek out this brown starfish. Many people are literally tight-assed. We walk around with the equivalent of a clenched fist in our pants. Then, when it's time to poop, we push so hard that tiny blood vessels pop, and hemorrhoids spring up like pimples on a rose. Once your rectum feels wrecked, it's understandable that some people write it off, like so much spilled milk. What can you do? In fact, your body is crying out to be noticed between these tight lips.

Seeing our anus is a great way to start reconnecting with this oft-neglected orifice. Suddenly, it's not a far away, abstract "other," but a loved part of our whole selves. So take some time to witness this innermost secret spot. You could light some candles to give it a feel of tenderness and intimacy. Or maybe put on a podcast and run the bath so everything feels totally normal, not weird at all, and

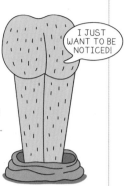

your roommates don't ask. Then stare down your brown eye in whatever way is comfortable for you. You might stand with a mirror behind you, bend over, look through your legs, and manually spread your cheeks. You could sit with bent, open legs and a mirror under your bottom. Lean back a bit, and you'll likely catch a glimpse of that little winker. Some have also found success squatting right over a mirror. If it's hard to see in real time, try using a phone camera on a timer, or ask a very close friend for a photo shoot. Just make sure it's a really good friend. Notice the shape of your anus. Its folds and wrinkles. Its hairstyle. Like a snowflake, each sphincter is unique and has different moods.

Throughout the day, mentally check in with your butthole. If you're clenching your asshole, you might be acting like one, too. Relax! You're not going to poop your pants. And when you do poop, be patient. Don't pressure yourself to push it out fast, but allow yourself to release. During cleanup, don't be afraid to get intimate with your anus. Especially if you have hemorrhoids or other irritation, a thorough and gentle cleaning with water or soft tissue is critical to restoring your healthy rear. Let's face it: if your anus ain't happy, ain't nobody happy. Butt love your anus, and your butt will love you back.

CHAPTER SIX

TOO DRY: CONSTIPATION

IT'S OFTEN BEEN SAID: WATER IS LIFE.
Landscapes ravaged by drought become brittle, cracked, and desolate of flourishing life. The same can roughly be said for your poop.

Many of us have experiential knowledge of constipation. Maybe we've been bloated, gassy, and cramping but can't seem to go. When we do finally get the urge, we push and strain, only to produce a tiny turdlet smaller than a sunflower seed. Constipation is not just physical; it can also take an emotional toll. It makes some people so irritable, they become ruthless dictators. Seriously! Hitler and Mussolini were reported to suffer regular constipation; it may even be part of what killed Napoleon. We know constipation in our bodies and minds; the term "constipation" refers to the physical experience of being clogged up. But the proof is in the pooping.

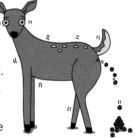

The poop that accompanies constipation might look rough and cracked. It could come out as a few little balls, like deer or sheep droppings. On the other hand, it could be painfully large painfully large and hard as a rock. Even if teeny tiny, it might feel somewhat sharp or painful coming out. Or it might not come out at all.

As you know, the Perfect Poop seems solid but is actually 75 percent water. Things are even wetter when digested food enters the large intestine. It's in this final go-round that the body takes its final slurp, absorbing water back into the body and leaving behind the spongy mass that will soon emerge as poop. When things get stuck in this stage, however, constipation occurs.

Of course, people don't generally decide to leave their undigested food hanging in the large intestine. Like so many things in the body, constipation results from complicated interactions between the body, mind, and external circumstances.

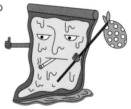

From a physiological perspective, constipation can be a sign that your insides are drying out. Perhaps you haven't had enough to drink, or the fluids you do imbibe are dehydrating (too much coffee and alcohol, for example). Proper hydration is required for basically everything in your body to function optimally, including digestion. When in doubt, drink more water. Once poop is in the picture, however, you're drinking for two.

A bulky, fibrous poo is much easier for your bowels to eliminate. Sure, the mucosal lining of your intestines and rectum gives slip to your stool's slide, but the peristaltic motion that pulses your poo into the world needs some cushion for the pushin'. That bulk is best supplied when non-digestible fiber from your diet soaks up and retains water like a sponge. So we can't simply hydrate ourselves into digestive health, we also need to consume a diet full of fiber-rich whole grains, fruits, and vegetables.

Imagine the way flour becomes bread with water, heat, and time. Your digestive tract is designed to offer optimal time in a hot oven. If your dough contains too much water compared to flour, however, it'll come out looking like goop. Too much flour compared to water, and it'll come out like bricks. With the appropriate ratios of water and fiber, your poop stays in the Goldiplops Zone and you pinch a perfect loaf.

Finding the perfect poo-dough recipe is your first line

of defense against becoming a constipated hard-ass. Again, that means consuming enough whole grains, vegetables, fruits, beans, etc., to supply your poop with bulky, absorbent fiber. And it means consuming enough water that, even once water is absorbed during the digestive process, there is still enough left to form a spongy poo. Oven time and temperatures vary, so the right ratios may be different for each person even under normal circumstances.

When circumstances become irregular, however, so do our bowels. Our digestion is strongly linked to our mental and emotional health. Sudden changes in our lives, whether small and temporary or big and permanent, can cause our systems to slow or shut down. Our bodies feel uncomfortable and insecure when we do. Being in a strange or new circumstance, like traveling to a new country or even staying at a friend's house, can leave our bowels feeling shy. We know that we should poop, we might even want to poop, but our bodies hold on for dear life. Unfortunately, constipation can be a self-fulfilling prophecy. The longer our bodies stay clogged up, the more water is drained from our stool, the harder our poop is to pass, and the longer we stay constipated.

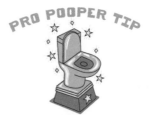

MOVE YOUR BODY, MOVE YOUR BOWELS

Mild constipation is often easily remedied with exercise. Just as emotional insecurity can manifest in our guts, our body's movements resonate in our bowels. Walk, jog, dance, or try yoga and gentle stretches to get (or keep) your digestive engine running smoothly. Remember how the large intestine winds up the right side of your abdomen, crosses to the left side under the ribs, and heads back down the left side toward your rectum? Sitting or lying in a twist, legs to the right and torso to the left, can help literally push the poo farther along its journey. Circular massage around the abdomen can have a similar effect.

In my own pooping experience, I've found that some movement can help even when on the toilet. Squatting is for sure the best way to poop in general, whether you use a stool to elevate your feet, perch on the seat, or adopt a toilet made for squatting. Assuming this position helps to open the puborectalis muscle, a sling that helps keep our rectums closed and our underpants clean while standing. Sitting at a ninety-degree angle opens it partway, but squatting or even leaning over your thighs can help to open it more fully.

Straining and bearing down too hard can cause hemorrhoids, rectal prolapse (when the walls of your rectum emerge through your anus; *shudder*), and even drain the blood from your head and cause you to pass out. Instead, push gently on your exhale and wiggle your body, like someone trying to get out of a tight dress. The poop is wiggling down and out, while your body is wriggling up and away. A hard or too-small stool may not have enough opposing friction, so that it winds up turtling in and out as you push and release. Try placing a few fingers around your anus, allowing that shy turdlet to slip out as you gently push your sphincter in the opposite direction. Then sigh in relief, and wash your hands with soap.

Sometimes we constipate ourselves through consciously not pooping. We've all been there. Nature calls, but we're not in a position to answer. Instead of going to voice mail, our poop heads back up the pike to wait. Now things get backed up as the water slowly drains out.

If we're lucky, we'll have another urge to poop when it's convenient, eliminate, and restore our natural cycles.

In an unlucky circumstance, we may try to return the call, but nature is nowhere to be found. Should this game of colon phone tag continue despite your valiant effort, things can quickly snowball. Or, more literally, shitball. We can wind up with a few days' worth of poo slowly accruing, drying out, and creating an ever larger and more difficult mass to pass.

Should this occur and your mailbox becomes completely full, take heart: once you do finally poop, your normal cycles should be quickly restored. One option is to simply wait until the urge to poop returns and, when it does, carpe doo-em! Do not wait! And don't overpush. Be patient and breathe as your butt slowly opens to birth the ungainly log. You can also help yourself along by taking natural fiber supplements (like psyllium husk, flax seeds, or prunes plus a lot of water), or the occasional laxative, stool softener, or enema. Be mindful that the body can become dependent on laxatives, so walk that middle path. Don't overuse them, but do take action within a few days if things begin to get backed up. Constipation can lead to impacted stool, which can require manual removal by a doctor. That would make quite an impact of its own, I'm sure.

Here's the bottom line: shit happens. It's okay! Do your best to eat well, stay hydrated, get exercise, and maintain mental wellness. And when constipation does happen, meet it with compassion. Your natural flow will often restore with just a little patience. If you do require greater intervention, be gentle with yourself. Remember that the mind and body are one thing; if you let constipation get you tense and tight, 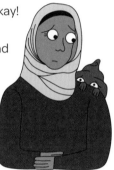 your bowels will really be in a bind. Relax. Stay loose! Your body doesn't want that shit in there any more than you do. Do your best to create the circumstances that promote easeful pooping, let go of the outcome, and know that your body will follow eventually.

CHAPTER SEVEN

TOO WET:
DIARRHEA

THE WORLD'S WATER is constantly cycling through the planet's systems. As an interconnected manifestation of the universe, the same is true for us. When not enough water is flowing, the planet's body experiences drought and our bodies suffer constipation. (And I do mean suffer . . .) When too much water is flowing, rivers overflow and so, too, do our bowels. We call this diarrhea.

The water in our bodies doesn't want to be bad. Its goal is to be absorbed or recycled. Water yearns to be sucked up through the intestinal walls and integrated into the cells. It fantasizes about being filtered by the kidneys and released back into the world as urine. It dreams of finding safe harbor in the strong arms of a high-fiber diet, where it can live as part of a bulky, firm stool before its happy ending in the toilet. Alas, not all dreams come to pass.

Poop becomes too dry when it stays in the body too long and too much water is absorbed. When food moves through too quickly, the body doesn't get to soak up those liquids, and poop comes out too wet. As with all things, wetness moves on a spectrum. The Perfect

Poop emerges like a scaly snake or a smooth banana.
A poo that's a little too wet cannot maintain its figure.
What can we say? It's let itself go.
Once upon a time, it had its shit
together. Now it comes out in
blobs and pieces.

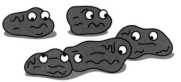

This semi-wet poo is a sign that you're getting plenty
of water, but not enough fiber for it to latch on to. It's
C-plus/ B-minus work. Because there is some fiber, you
can see distinct pieces of poo in the bowl. But instead of
your body forming a nice, solid corn on the cob, you're
staring down a rag tag smattering of popcorn. If this is
what's revealed in your crystal bowl, try reducing your
reliance on processed foods and animal products, and
eat more whole plants. Like fresh-popped
popcorn! A few handfuls and you'll poop
like a valedictorian.

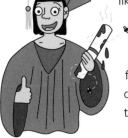

Blobs in the toilet can also mean
you're drinking too much coffee or alcohol. I know, I know. You
can't have any fun, can you? But
the key is really about moderation.

You probably know from your own body that coffee gets things moving, and your younger self remembers what the toilet bowl would look like after a night of heavy drinking. It's not pretty. That's because both of these liquids stimulate and dehydrate; they get water moving out. And that means out your butt. Slow things down by countering those espresso or tequila shots with tall glasses of water, and maybe a slice of prune. Shaken, not stirred.

Further along the wetness spectrum, things start to get really sloppy. We're talking mushy porridge, chunky smoothie, or eerily silky-smooth liquid. The technical 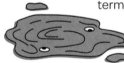 term is "diarrhea," but the ridiculous state in which it leaves the sufferer has made it the stuff of children's songs and silly names: "the trots," "Hershey squirts," "Montezuma's revenge." This poo is hard to hold back; any weakness in the sphincter's tight grip could lead to leakage. It often comes out explosively and urgently, making grown men cry and hold their butts. This poo earns its nickname "the runs" both for the way it finds us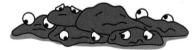

sprinting to the bathroom and how the contents of our bowels race out of us.

Diarrhea is a sign that something is not working. Under ideal circumstances, your meal would move slowly through the intestines so that water, nutrients, and electrolytes can be absorbed. In this case, your body is rushing things through as fast as it can. That means it's not absorbing all that good stuff, which is really bad. Recurrent diarrhea can lead to dehydration and even malnutrition. Rather than passing go and collecting $200, diarrhea runs the red light and robs the bank.

Diarrhea is the anal equivalent to vomiting—a comparison that in itself might make you feel queasy. In general, stomach irritation causes vomiting. Irritation farther down in the intestines likely leads to diarrhea. But what irritant is to blame? Who is this Montezuma, and why does he want revenge? (I'll give you a hint! #Colonialism.)

Diarrhea is the result of complex interactions between our food, circumstances, mind, and body, same as constipation. That 11:00 p.m. sushi? It's 50 percent off because it might go through you in half the time. Bad bugs can develop and hitch a ride into our system on undercooked or under-refrigerated foods. If diarrhea hasn't abated in a day or two, see a medical professional who may be able to help diagnose what's going on.

Many bacteria are harmless, or even beneficial, and we can develop some immunity or symbiosis to microorganisms in our normal environment. Encounters with foreign bugs, however, can lead to what's commonly called "traveler's diarrhea," regardless of how "developed" the country or sanitary the circumstances. Hence, Montezuma was not bothered by the microorganisms that now plague visitors to Aztec lands. But any Aztec person drinking from my tap—and thus downing the unfamiliar E. coli in the water—might similarly get the squirts.

Diarrhea can also be the result of poop bugs being where they shouldn't. We tend to call this "food poisoning," but the problem actually resides with the fecal bacteria hitchhiking on your hoagie. Maybe manure was applied to leafy greens before the fertilizer was fully processed and safe, or the lettuce it went on was not washed thoroughly. Or maybe you didn't wash your hands after pooping, and then cooked what might have been remembered as a lovely wedding banquet if all the guests hadn't soiled their undies. Smokey says, "Only you can prevent forest fires." I say, "Only you can prevent fecal fires." Please, folks, wash your hands with soap.

Food can be a carrier for problematic pathogens, but it can also be the problem itself. We hear a lot these days about wheat sensitivity, for example, and experts estimate that over 65 percent of the world's population has negative reactions to lactose from dairy. (As my friend Elvi used to say, "I will not tolerate lactose!")

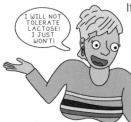

If you think you might be sensitive to certain foods, try keeping a log log (see page 31) and look for a correlation between what comes in and what comes out. Notice what happens when you eliminate potential triggers, go on a low-FODMAP (fermentable oligosaccharides, disaccharides, monosaccharides, and polyols, aka short-chain carbohydrates) diet, reinforce your microbiome with fermented foods, or follow the advice of a trusted health and nutrition professional. Don't give up hope! Some people find that their guts can be rehabilitated over time, and they can slowly bring old favorites back without overflowing the banks of their bowels.

Stress eating is another way food can bring us short term relief on the "in" and watery regret on the "out." When stressed, we often reach for sugary, fatty, highly processed foods that irritate our system, especially in large quantities. Not that I or my friends Ben, Jerry, and Jack Daniel's know anything about this . . .

In fact, the same anxiety and stress that earlier plugged us up, at other times can fling the floodgates wide open. Yes, as part of our "fight-or-flight" response, we literally can be scared shitless. But the gut's response to stress is actually much more nuanced than that and, for some people, much more persistent. Our bowels are tethered to our central nervous system and also have their own internal sensory network called the enteric system. You could say that the mind and gut are intricately connected, but that misrepresents the fact that they operate as one unified entity. The brain is a digestive organ; our digestive system thinks and feels. We are thinking, feeling, digesting beings.

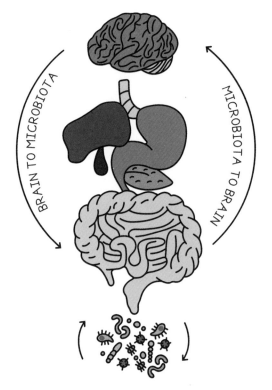

MICROBIAL DIVERSITY + RELATIVE ABUNDANCE

This gut response evolved over millions of years to help us navigate a sometimes stressful world. That's good, and we benefit from this in moments of peak tension. But our world has evolved much faster than we have and, in an ironic twist of lime, left our behinds behind. Many of us have it better than it's ever been, yet we're chronically stressed, uneasy, and racked with doubt. Chronic diarrhea is just the symptom; Montezuma's real revenge is the ever-present fear and insatiable desire that blankets contemporary life.

The best thing you can do for anxious, chronic diarrhea? Relax. Take care of yourself. Practice being in the moment, rather than replaying the past or worrying about the future. The best antidote to anxiety is to appreciate your life right now, exactly as it is. Therapy is good, too. And if that fails, see my friends Ben, Jerry, and Jack—in moderation, of course.

Here's the bottom line: shit happens! It's okay. Do your best to eat fresh and clean food, get plenty of fiber, and invest in your mental wellness. And when wet poops happen, or you really get the trots, sally forth with compassion and stay close to the toilet. With a healthy immune system, minor disturbances should clear up in a few days. Drink plenty of water and electrolytes in the meantime. If things don't solidify after that, stay calm but pay attention. Your body is trying to tell you something. Listen to the liquid burbling out of your butt, and

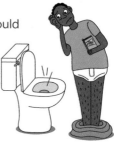

consult a professional you trust. Most importantly, align yourself with peace, ease, and justice in the world. Right former wrongs, live without shame, and the spirit of Montezuma might just bless your bowels.

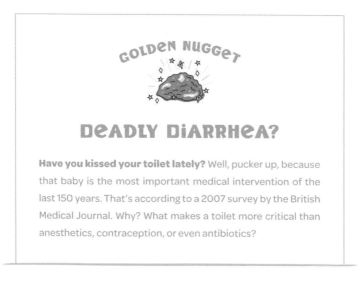

GOLDEN NUGGET

DEADLY DIARRHEA?

Have you kissed your toilet lately? Well, pucker up, because that baby is the most important medical intervention of the last 150 years. That's according to a 2007 survey by the British Medical Journal. Why? What makes a toilet more critical than anesthetics, contraception, or even antibiotics?

As you know, when fecal bacteria make it into our mouths, diarrhea can result. But that's just the tip of the turd-berg. Diseases like cholera, hepatitis, giardia, parasites like tapeworm, and many, many more nasty inflictions can all spread from poop. The key is to quarantine that crap from the moment of deposit until it can be processed, treated, rendered harmless, and even become beneficial.

Unfortunately, an estimated 2.4 to 3.6 billion people—almost half the global population, including millions in the US—still don't have a safe and sanitary toilet. This means poop gets out into the world, makes people very sick, and—VERY SAD FACT WARNING—kills children. According to UNICEF in 2021, "Every day, over 700 children under age 5 die from diarrhea linked to unsafe water, sanitation, and poor hygiene." While already tragic, this figure does not account for the time and prosperity lost due to sickness, expensive care and medicines, or the permanent stunting from malnutrition common for those suffering chronic diarrhea due to lack of sanitation. In some countries, these losses can equal up to 6 percent GDP. That's some expensive shit! Adding insult to critical injury, because this crisis involves the taboo topics of poop and toilets, the world often ignores this issue or deals with it under the euphemism of "waterborne diseases."

Major bummer, right?

But there is good news. The world is slowly waking up to this most-unsexy crisis. While the United Nations left sanitation off the Millennium Development Goals set in 2000, it was added in 2002 and has since become a major priority as part of the Sustainable Development Goals for 2030. Increased attention from philanthropy, social entrepreneurs, and governments across the world has lent much-needed urgency, funds, and innovation to this crisis. Because basic sanitation is at the foundation of any healthy society, the returns are enormous; every dollar invested in water and sanitation returns at least $4 in money saved.

Looking to doo some good in the world? Give a shit, go online, and drop some cash to an organization working for change. Together, we can ensure that everyone has a toilet to smooch.

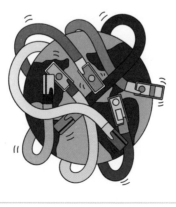

CHAPTER EIGHT

JUST RIGHT: THE GOLDIPLOPS ZONE

THE ELUSIVE PERFECT POOP. It's so close, I can taste it! Ew . . . um, actually, let's just take a look instead.

Not too dry, and not too wet, the Perfect Poop splashes down in the Goldiplops Zone. Sometimes smooth like a snake, and sometimes gently riddled with cracks, this sausage-like beauty (numbering one or a few links) could almost slip out unnoticed. Its size may impress you, even while scoring extra points from your end zone for its easy release. This shit sails so smoothly it might not need much cleanup, and is so full of fiber it might even float. The smell, too, is better than the average BM. Like Mary Poopins, it's practically perfect in every way.

As you already know, any poo that comes out of you is a complex amalgamation of your mind, body, circumstances, and the food you ate. All poos contain the same basic ingredients: mostly water, a lot of gut bacteria and fiber, and some undigested proteins, fats, and minerals. The Perfect Poop requires a recipe with ideal ingredient ratios from the food and beverages you consume. Just as importantly, it requires a centered chef with access to adequate time and a few basic tools. You do not have to be a saint to experience holy shit, but too much sin will definitely throw you off.

Let's start with food. If you've been reading from the beginning, you know that hitting the Goldiplops Zone means forging a strong bond between water and fiber inside your body. Too much fiber, not enough water, and you're going to feel stuck up. Too dry! Too much water, not enough fiber, and you'll be in the splash zone. Too wet!

Unfortunately, I can't tell you what the proper ratios are for you; it's different for everybody. Some people's systems can do a lot with a little, while others are much more fragile and easily stray from the path. The only way to know is by paying attention to what you eat, what you poop, and getting to know your shit.

That said, most people will see the greatest benefit from eating a consistent diet of plant-centered, whole foods and drinking lots of water. The dietary fibers your colon craves are not naturally found in meat or dairy

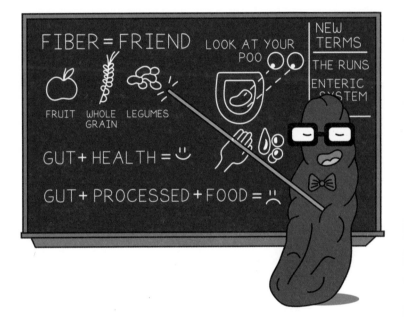

products and have often been extracted from packaged, processed foods. Even minimally processed plant foods, like fruit juice, are often bereft of the fibrous pulp with which fresh fruit furnishes your feces. Fiber supplements can also help, but they cannot replace the many added benefits of getting your fiber from real, honest-to-goodness food. Hey, if it's the only way you're willing to get fiber, then go for it. Live your dreams! But I would encourage most people to bulk up on fruits, veggies, whole grains, nuts, legumes, beans, and all the wonders of the garden whenever you can.

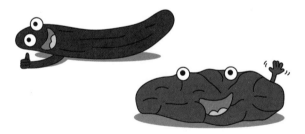

Ultimately, look to your poo. It's the expert when it comes to your body. If what you're doing is working, the Perfect Poop will appear. If not, thank your body! It's giving you valuable information. Take the hint, go back to the cutting board, and try again tomorrow.

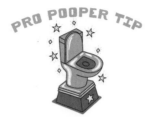

FEED YOUR FECES

Looking for easy ways to bulk up on fiber? Any whole plant food can help, but pound per pound, these foods really pack a poopy punch:

- Raspberries
- Avocados
- Blackberries
- Artichokes
- Lentils
- Split peas
- Kidney beans
- Chickpeas

- Bulgur
- Oats
- Popcorn (my favorite, air-popped with a little oil, salt, and nutritional yeast!)
- Almonds
- Pistachios
- Sunflower seeds

Bowels in a bind? Chia seeds and ground flaxseeds are nature's fiber supplements. Try adding a spoonful or two into cereals, smoothies, and yogurt, on salads, or just about anywhere you can sneak them. You can also mix a spoonful or two with water and drink it down as a supplement. Just be careful: these thirsty seeds will soak up water in your body and make for powerful poo. To keep your ratios right, be sure to drink a lot more water, or things will get dry and seedy.

The Perfect Poop cannot live on whole-grain bread alone. Even when eating an ideal diet, stress and anxiety can throw your shit directly into the fan. As you know, the gut and the brain are intricately connected—we are one, unified organism. Stress in the mind cannot help but manifest as stress in the body, and vice versa.

The beautiful thing about this mind-body non-duality is that we can exert influence on our whole being from either side of the equation. If we notice anxious thoughts, we can work with them directly through meditation or journaling, or we can direct ourselves out of our minds by working with our bodies. If we notice tension creeping into our muscles, we can take a bath, do some yoga, or redirect our attention toward mindfulness. It doesn't really matter which side of the seesaw you play on, what's important is that you stay in balance and have fun.

Like that seesaw, we find our balance through movement, change, and constant rebalancing. No one is going to be blissed out and Zen all of the time, and if they are, they're probably a dog.

One of the best things we can do is to release ourselves from that expectation and embrace the inevitability of some discomfort, and the reality of constant flow. Doing that, we can stop trying to hold on to any particular state and, instead, simply regulate as needed. Magically, however, the more we practice self-care and integrate it into our everyday lives, the harder it is for things to take us way off balance.

It's a mindful oxymoron: worry over whether you have your shit together, and shit will most definitely fall apart. Go with the flow, and the Perfect Poop is more likely to appear.

CHILL OUT, SQUAT DOWN, GIVE UP CONTROL

Maintaining our overall health and social-emotional wellness is fundamental to aiming for the Goldiplops Zone. That means getting adequate sleep and exercise, eating fresh foods and drinking plenty of water, and recharging with community and through self-care. Once you've done all that good work, don't leave it at the bathroom door! Take it with you to the toilet, and move your bowels mindfully. Pooping is a practical act, but it's also an opportunity to be in close communion with your body. (For many parents and people pooping at work, it's also one of the few times you might get a minute to yourself!)

No, you don't have to chant "om" as you poop, unless that boats your floaters. But how can your time in the restroom be an extension of self-care, love, and, well, rest? Studies show that you're going to spend anywhere from fifteen minutes to an hour in the bathroom every day. Make it count! Invest in creating a warm, cozy environment and, more importantly, a loving inner landscape that can help coax that crap right out of you.

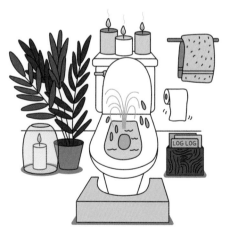

Maybe you think I'm off my squatter, but a Perfect Poo should come out almost effortlessly. If you're pushing and straining, you're working too hard. (And you're probably still sitting; see page 74 as to why you should adopt a squatting posture.) Sure, sometimes we have to squeeze one out between meetings, but all that tension in your sphincter will make even the most well-formed stool come out looking like spaghetti. Relax. Release! Listen to your body's natural rhythms, keep breathing, and let your anus and pelvic floor open as your abdominal muscles help move things down and out. Aren't you glad you lightened your load?

SHiT TO GOLD: THe POO-LOSOPHeR'S STONe

Like a Russian nesting doll, our world is composed of systems within systems, connected through a series of ins and out. As I write, my body eats and poops inside a house, which itself takes resources from the urban environment and pumps or trucks waste back out. The urban system feeds from and dumps into its regional ecology, which, in turn, consumes, digests, and excretes like one organ of the interconnected earth body. As long as everything stays in balance, all poops become food, and no one suffocates on their own shit.

Unfortunately, our supersized lifestyles have pushed earth's systems way off balance, almost to their breaking point. I won't go into the specifics because, unless you're living in a cave with your fingers in your ears, you already know and suffer sleepless nights because of it. One of the biggest engines driving us into the abyss is our consumer culture. As far as most economists are concerned, that's our identity: "consumers." And like a giant mouth, we unwittingly follow suit, glorifying shopping, celebrating food, and gobbling up media.

Numerous studies show, however, that all this intake isn't making us happier. Instead, we wind up constipated: shelves, closets, and basements filled with crap we don't need. The rest runs right through us like diarrhea, without offering any nutrition in return. In fact, a full 99 percent of what goes through our systems of mass production is trash within six months. Astounding, right? In order to keep the myth of infinite consumption alive, we're taught to ignore our output. What comes out is covered over, carted away, flushed, forgotten "waste."

But there is no "away" in a closed-loop system; we're like a flatulent man under the covers, slowly choking on our own gas.

Poop reminds us that there is another way. Sure, we are consumers by nature. But we're also creators, producers, POOPERS! Our bodies know how to live in harmony with the planet, taking in the resources we need, and furnishing the earth with resources in return. In fact, enough nutrients come back out in your pee and poo to grow your food all over again. The fertilizer in your urine, for example, could grow enough wheat to make a loaf of bread every single day. We're basically pooping prosperity! We have more than enough; we just can't keep using more than we have.

CONCLUSION

EAT.
POOP.
LOVe.

CONGRATULATIONS, DEAR POOPER! You've made it to the tail end. You are getting to know your shit, and are well on your way to excremental excellence.

Even as we strive for ever more Perfect Poop, it's important to remember: shit isn't good or bad. And we don't want to fix poop for poop's sake; it's just a piece of shit! We want to fix poop for our literal selves, for our bodies. The Perfect Poop tells us that our particular combination of mind and body, food and circumstances, is working together to provide an optimal human experience. That's not a static target. Some days are more stressful, and some are chill. Sometimes we feel healthy, and sometimes we're ill. We might nourish mindfully on Monday, and then celebrate with pizza, wings, and beer on Friday. Great! Live your life! The most important thing is to know what optimal and "regular" means for you so you can identify when your poop is trying to pull you back on the path.

The Perfect Poop isn't something outside ourselves for which we have to struggle and strive. It's already inside you. It is you! Poop becomes perfected not because of its fiber content, diverse gut microbes, or even your relaxed rectum. It's the care and attention you devote to your doo that allows your turd to transcend. It's the love and respect with which you listen to your load that allows that load to love you back. By giving a crap about crap, you get to know your shit, and learn to love yourself from the bottom up. The rest is details.

Thanks so much for reading. I hope this book has brought you relief. May it be for the benefit of your bowels and for the greater happiness of all beings. Poop in peace.

BiO

Shawn Shafner (he/they) is an artist, educator, and facilitator. As founder of The People's Own Organic Power (POOP) Project, Shawn catalyzes conversations about sustainable sanitation for every pooper—and the planet we poop on. From the floor of the United Nations to the mountains of Rwanda, he has spread poop positivity since 2010 on four continents, at colleges across the country, toured four critically-acclaimed shows, released three years of podcast episodes, produced one feature-length documentary, and had countless conversations about the doo we all do doo. More at thePOOPproject.org. When he's not pooping, Shawn teaches meditation and mindful creativity, leads movement classes through the lineage of choreographer Tamar Rogoff, sings with Marisa Michelson's Constellation Chor Ensemble, tells stories to young children and their families, and facilitates arts-integrated workshops for learners of all ages. Shawn is the humble recipient of some fancy fellowships, grants, and awards. His work is featured in three books (now four!), and he's performed at Madison Square Garden, with the New York Philharmonic at Lincoln Center, and many more—but he doesn't like to brag. He just wants to spread love, have fun, and make meaningful connections. So let's get started already!

ShawnShafner.com

ABOUT CiDER MiLL PRESS BOOK PUBLiSHERS

Good ideas ripen with time. From seed to harvest, Cider Mill Press brings fine reading, information, and entertainment together between the covers of its creatively crafted books. Our Cider Mill bears fruit twice a year, publishing a new crop of titles each spring and fall.

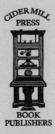

"Where Good Books Are Ready for Press"

Visit us online at
cidermillpress.com
or write to us at
PO Box 454
12 Spring St.
Kennebunkport, Maine 04046

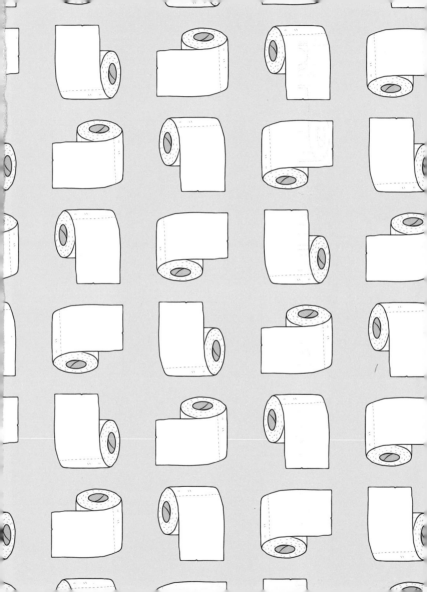

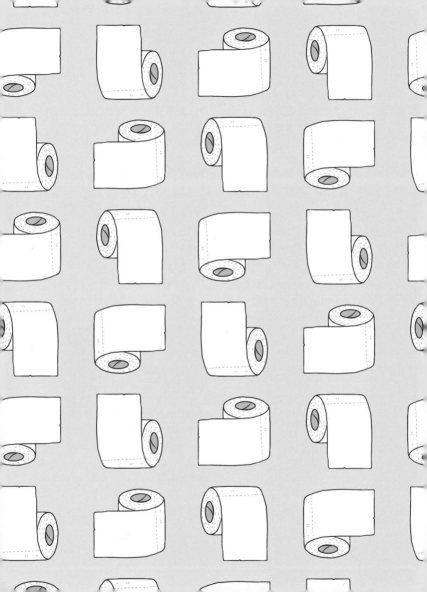